Have a meeting with yourself ... be ready to design the life you love. Focus on the contents of this *Guide* more than you would on decorating your dream home. We devote a lot of attention to the place where we live while in fact we should be focusing on the life we lead!

Working with this *Guide*, you will:
- Build your internal peace
- Discover the pleasure of being yourself and knowing your worth
- Get to know yourself and then see what in your life only needs renovation and what you should tear down or abandon to find happiness
- Focus on yourself and your needs.

How many times have you criticized your life?

How many times have others made fun of your decisions?

How many times have you given up and abandoned your dream for fear of ridicule?

Time to end it. Now is your time.

Congratulations on your decision to change!

I'm going to help you understand what values matter in your life. You decide what to do next. I'm going to show you the way and if you want, you will be able to follow it and I will proudly watch you bravely march forward.

I can prepare you for a change if you give me 30 minutes a day for the next 21 days. The power is with you! You are the architect of your life!

I wish you good luck discovering yourself!
Kasia Dorosz

Spis treści

Introduction 3
Your daily plan 3
    Morning ritual 3
    Evening ritual 5
    Tasks for the next 21 days 5
1. My happy morning 7
2. A journey inside yourself 9
3. Love and happiness in your home 11
4. Inspirations 13
5. Traveling 15
6. A sense of happiness 17
7. Your talents 19
8. Acceptance 21
9. Your inner strength 23
10. Who is important to you? 27
11. A happy person's litany 29
12. The need for love and the language of love according to Chapman 33
13. Your inner critic 37

Copyright © 2019 Katarzyna Dorosz

No part of this publication may be reproduced, stored in a retrieval system, or transmitted in any form or by any means, electronic, mechanical, photocopied, recorded, scanned without the prior written permission of the author.

Introduction

Independent of the other volumes, the *Guide* you are holding in your hands is to be a signpost towards a road full of peace. However, the following information remains the same for the entire series.

To work with the *Guide* you will need:

1. An exercise book
Write in it the answers to all the questions that I ask you in individual tasks for each given day.

2. A book calendar
Use it to summarise your days.

Your daily plan

Remember to start and end each day with gratitude, meditation and exercises. At this stage, you can now adjust their duration and order to your needs. My suggestion is as follows:

Morning ritual

1. Gratitute and affirmations
Focus on the good that surrounds you. Say aloud what you are grateful for. Make some positive statements about yourself.

2. Reading and meditation
Read some quotes, the Holy Bible or a valuable book. Choose one thought from the text that will guide you through the day. Then sit back and contemplate it for a few minutes. Finally, focus on your breath, put all thoughts away and remain silent for a few moments.

3. Exercises
Do a few simple exercises – move your body to start a good day.

Evening ritual

1. **A recap of your day and gratitude**

   In your book calendar, please write the answers to the following questions:

   What am I grateful for today? What good did I do today? What have I learned today? How much did I practice today? What did I eat today?

2. **Relaxation exercises**

   Do some stretching exercises to get rid of tensions that arose in your body during the day.

3. **Meditation**

   Find a comfortable position to contemplate in. Calm your thoughts. Focus on your breath. Release everything that happened throughout the day from your mind.

Tasks for the next 21 days

Focus on reading a fragment of the text assigned for every day. Determine the time of day when you can work on it in peace and quiet – do it diligently and in sequence.

Think about what your life has been like so far and how you want it to be. What do you need to do to achieve it? Write all your ideas in your workbook. The next day, read that text carefully and go for a half-hour walk alone. While you walk, other ideas for change are sure to cross your mind. Note them down in your notebook and start implementing them one by one.

Workbook 4

Your Guide to Positive Life

1. MY HAPPY MORNING

Every morning, when you wake up and open your eyes, let the first thought be gratitude. Give thanks for everything you have – for your health, food, shelter, for every little thing in your life.

Then massage your kidneys, liver and heart. Think with tenderness about your internal organs. Send them love: „I love you, my heart" – listen to how it beats for you.

Sit comfortably on the floor and indulge in peaceful contemplation of your feelings and thoughts. Focus on your breathing.

Be present in the moment
Now take a book of quotes or prayers. Read the previously prepared passage. When you feel inner peace get up and joyfully start your wonderful day!

Exercise 1:
Find a source of daily inspiration – go to a library or bookstore and find a book there that you can use every morning. Make sure it contains sentences worth thinking over to enrich your life.

Exercise 1I:
Every day, consider the next parts of the book.
Write down in your book calendar:
1. What does the passage you've read mean to you?
2. How has it changed your life?

Morning readings are meant to not only be a pleasure, but above all an incentive to look inside yourself and an incentive to change.

Your Guide to Positive Life

2. A JOURNEY INSIDE YOURSELF

You are the creator of your reality. If you want it to be beautiful, then make it so. **Your life is the mirror of your soul**. Nothing matters as much as YOU do.

Your life,
Your body,
Your thoughts,
Happiness
are what matters!

Repeat it to yourself every day. With love and respect – you are the most important to yourself. You have control over your life. You create your reality the way you want it to be.

There is nothing greater than true love. **The first person you will love is you yourself.** Is it hard? Very hard.

It often happens that we start looking for something external in our lives, something that is not there. The first rule is: start with yourself, look for it in yourself. You are YOUR OWN master! **Remember that you are whoever you decide to become**.

Exercise 1:

Ask yourself the following questions and write down your answers in the workbook:

1. What do I want to improve from my past? What can I influence and what can I change?
2. What do I want to consciously preserve from my past?
3. What I hate and how to end it?
4. What steps do I need to take to start these changes here and now?
5. Do I have everything I need? If not, what am I missing to achieve my goals?

Exercise II:

What story from the book is close to your heart? What character or type of chaacter? How would you like to be similar to this hero? Remember, you are the lead character of the story of your life.

Your Guide to Positive Life

3. LOVE AND HAPPINESS IN YOUR HOME

Bring joy into your home. It is said that the home is made by the people who create it. It is possible that now the only person who creates your home is you. Both the death of a spouse and the departure of children from home are associated with a sense of mourning. Elisabeth Kübler-Ross, an American doctor, has distinguished three components of mourning: loss, longing and feeling lost. They are all difficult, but you will manage to overcome each of them, and when the time comes – to bring joy to your home.

Exercise I:
Close your eyes, take a deep breath and exhale, calm your mind and think:
- What brings you joy?
- What makes you feel free?
- Who do you feel happy with?

Record all your thoughts in the workbook.

Exercise II:
To bring joy to your home, you may need to make some small changes. During my lectures I often hear stories of people who devote their whole lives to helping others. It's beautiful. At the same time, if you are one of these people, it's time to take care of yourself and your surroundings too!

Consider:
1. What do you love about your home? View? Memories? Colors?
2. What annoys you at home or makes you lose your life energy? A cluttered room? Dirty walls – maybe it's time to think about a minor renovation that will make you wake up in the morning.

I don't know if you are aware of it, but a small thing such as the color of the walls has a huge impact on you! The bedroom should be in subdued and soft colors to facilitate sleep, and the room dedicated to your daily work and entertainment should preferably be in a bright and joyful color. **Think what and when you can change in your home so that it can bring you more joy.**

Your Guide to Positive Life

4. INSPIRATIONS

All of us need inspiration, authorities and role models – someone who will show us how to achieve happiness in our lives, but also how to maintain it.

Many people have an impact on your life. The people you meet in your everyday environment – family, friends, random people you meet while shopping in the store. You can also observe the lives of famous people, admire historical figures or marvel at fictional literary characters whose actions are close to your heart.

Remember!
You can draw from many sources. One person may be your inspiration in terms of a healthy lifestyle, and another may impress you with their persistence in the face of difficulties.

Exercise:
Now think about the people you admire and who inspire you. Write their names in your workbook, and then write the answers to the following questions next to each name:
1. What do I admire this person for?
2. What about their behavior do I want to add to my life?
3. What role do they play in my life?
4. Can I have a closer relationship with them? If so, how can I do it?

It is important that you realize why you admire and like other people. It reveals the important truth about you as a human being – it shows what you want in your life. In addition, conscious analysis of your inspirations will make you look at the people around you with more gratitude and love: the next step to achieve joy and peace of mind.

Your Guide to Positive Life

5. TRAVELING

We all love traveling, although we all have different preferences for our travels. Some love visiting new fascinating places, discovering new cultures and meeting new people. Others are happy traveling alone in the mountains or organizing short sightseeing trips with their loved ones.

It is said that travel educates and there is a lot of truth in it that is worth considering.

Exercise I:
Think about how you like to travel. What type of rest brings you real peace and relaxation? What places do you like to visit? Do you prefer traveling alone or do you need a companion to share your experiences? If you like traveling in company, who do you like to travel with the most?

Exercise II:
1. Now, are there any places you would like to see? The ones you haven't visited yet or you remember them such fondness that you would like to go back again? Write down the closest and the farthest one away from you.
2. Think about what you need to do to make your dream come true - check everything in detail, as if you were going there now. Among others, check how to get there. What would you like to see there? How much time would you like to spend there? How much would the whole trip cost you? Remember what you worked on in the previous exercise – your favorite way of traveling.
3. Now you know exactly what your dream looks like, so... start making it come true! Create a plan – these are just two trips, start implementing them in turn. Where will you start?

What gives me a sense of peace is the feeling of making my dreams come true. Now you can feel it too.

Your Guide to Positive Life

6. A SENSE OF HAPPINESS

Be kind to yourself. Respect yourself, your thoughts and feelings. Pay attention to how you approach people. This is a mirror – it shows who you are and what your values are, but your behavior is also reflected in other people – when you are kind, others are the same. Give as much love and respect as you can bear. **Be a giver of happiness – and it will return to you multiplied.**

I know what some of you may think: „I am kind to people and they throw logs under my feet". Remember that these are the exceptions! Think about it, maybe it's time to end your relationship with them – cut yourself off from toxic people and don't make your sense of happiness dependent on them.

Stop for a moment and see how delicate a butterfly is – a beautiful creature, right? You are beautiful and delicate too.

Look inwards now. What do you feel and see? Beauty? Sensitivity? Kindness? Yes, that's YOU.

Feel it – treat yourself and your body as the most beautiful temple. Like the most refined diamonds!

Exercise I:
Can you laugh spontaneously and from the bottom of your heart? Create your own list of people, places, things or activities that make you happy. Let this be your happiness list.

Exercise II:
Take a close look at the four aspects of your life:
1. Emotional – write down the feelings you have for yourself and others; highlight the ones you want to work on,
2. Intellectual – consider what you think about yourself and the people you meet. What needs changing?
3. Physical – what does your body say to you? Do you show it love and respect?
4. Spiritual – what do you believe in and how do you apply your faith to your everyday life?

Your Guide to Positive Life

7. YOUR TALENTS

Each of us has skills that we can work on throughout our lives. For some it is dance, for others it is singing, painting, knitting, crocheting, cooking... There are many possibilities and it is never too late to discover your talent and enjoy it.

Remember!

Just because you're over fifty doesn't mean you can't, for example, start playing the violin. Give up the belief that if you do something, you need to master it to perfection and be the best. You don't! Act for the pleasure of creative life.

Exercise I:

Write down what you are good at. What is your secret weapon? What hidden strength and power lies within you?

Exercise II:

Take the time to think about what activities you have enjoyed so far in your life. What would you like to try? What would you like to learn? Think about several possible talents:

1. Artistic – painting, drawing, clay moulding, etc. Maybe you would like to visit art galleries and exhibitions?
2. Musical – singing, playing an instrument (which one?), composing, dancing, etc. Maybe you like going to concerts and can't imagine a home without music?
3. Sports – is movement the necessary part of your life? What physical activity do you like to do the most?
4. Literary – writing a diary or journal, poems and stories, etc.
5. Technical – constructing new devices, improving the space around you, repairing and renovating objects – maybe that's something you like?
6. Others – I have listed only a few popular talent groups to help guide you towards what you can do in your life. However, there are many more. Find what your strengths are and develop them.

Your Guide to Positive Life

8. ACCEPTANCE

A happy person accepts everything that happens to them. They understands that life is a lesson which lets them acquire new knowledge, skills and experience.

They take full responsibility for their life – they know that it is up to them whether they take advantage of opportunities and how they react to random misfortunes and unexpected problems.

A person accepting reality is absolutely not passive and submissive. They know that by accepting everything they gain the power that will allow them to shape reality according to their own wishes. They can achieve peace and happiness regardless of external conditions.

Exercise I:
Are you that kind of person?
Think about the things you find difficult to accept. List them all. Think about the reason for the lack of acceptance, because only knowing that will you be able to change it.

Exercise II:
When saying „acceptance" we often want to add „self" before it – and rightly so, as it is very important! To achieve it, first of all, you need to get to know yourself, so think about:
1. What is most important to you as a human?
2. What do you like about yourself the most?
3. Is there anyone in your life who believes in you more than you do? Who is it? How do you feel about what they say about you?

Exercise III:
Uncover and accept your past!
1. What do you regret in your life?
2. What have you never managed to get done?
3. What does this change in you? How would it help you change yourself and who you are?

Your Guide to Positive Life

9. YOUR INNER STRENGTH

External factors cannot dictate how you feel or how you behave. Although giving up the control of your life to fate or other people can bring peace, that peace is only superficial! It weakens you, makes you become someone you really aren't and ultimately leads to a gap between your needs and desires and the compulsion to conform to someone else's vision. If that is what your life looks like, it's time to change it. How? By discovering your inner strength!

Exercise I:

Open up to your feelings and emotions – they are a reliable compass indicating things that build you up and those that stand in the way of your happiness. Every day after morning meditation, answer these questions:

1. What do I feel? - stop at different moments of your day and listen to what your emotions and body tell you. Keep in touch with yourself.
2. Do you feel respect for yourself?
3. Do you feel that you have good intentions in life?
4. How do you feel about the people you meet every day? Do you feel that everything is clear to everyone and you don't have to hide anything?

Remember to always keep your intentions, actions and feelings pure. When you do this, you will achieve peace – internal stability. Too often do I see people who are ashamed of their own desires and decisions. It wears them out because although they want to do something, they try to hide it from the general public for fear of the reaction they might meet with. Do you feel how much anxiety this may cause? Don't do this to yourself! Although it is very difficult at first, do everything to act openly – proud of yourself and of what you do.

Exercise II:

Build your inner strength and peace by learning who you are deep inside. Consider and write down the answers to the following questions:
1. What is more important to you than knowledge?
2. What is more powerful than death?
3. What leads you to be strong every day?
4. Do you have inner peace? If so, how is it expressed? If not, write down why and what could you do to achieve it.

Exercise III:

Write an evaluation of your life. You can do it in two ways:
1. Divide your life into stages, e.g. childhood, adolescence, family building and work experience, second youth (life from your fifties on!). Then make a table for each period and write at least five examples of:

Your most valued memories	The most difficult situations you lived through	People and things that were important to you	Mistakes that you made	Lessons that you learnt

Finally, write a short summary of each stage of your life.

2. Use your imagination and think about what you would compare your life to.
„My life is like a poem ...", „My life is like music ...", „My life is like a butterfly in the wind ...", „My life is like a circus ..."

Exercise IV:

Now that you have a full picture of your past, focus on the future. List ten things you would like to accomplish. Feel the power of imagination!

Workbook 4

Your Guide to Positive Life

10. WHO IS IMPORTANT TO YOU?

A happy person loves and accepts themselves. They have the right amount of self-esteem because they know their own value. They know that all the seemingly negative situations they have experienced in their life were only sources of experience. Of course, they accept their imperfections and work on them.

A person who loves themselves has so much love that they begin to give it to other people. They share it and radiate it. Only by truly and unconditionally loving ourselves can we really and unconditionally love others.

Exercise I:
If you were to spend the whole year with only one person, who would it be? Pay equal attention to who did not appear in your thoughts and why – such a simple exercise shows a lot about relationships that need healing.

Exercise II:
Now please write down the names of the people you rejected in the previous exercise.
How much energy can you spend on changing your relationships with these people? What would have to change for you to spend the whole year with them with pleasure?

Exercise III:
Now write ten sentences about the person who is closest to you. Focus on who they are and what makes them so important to you. When was the last time you told a loved one how you felt about them and how important they are to you?
Can you listen to them actively and talk to them honestly?

Exercise IV:
Write down the five things you wish to your loved ones. Think about what they would wish for and not what you think is best for them.

Your Guide to Positive Life

11. A HAPPY PERSON'S LITANY

Be in the moment
The present is the timelessness of existence.
By being in the moment, we overcome time and aging.
Stop thinking about the past and the future. Live the present! Someone once calculated that an average person devotes only about 1 minute every day to the present, the rest consists of plans and memories. By being present in the moment we see details that we would not have noticed by focusing on the past and the future.

Eat mindfully
It is best to be in tune with the real needs of the body. Conscious nutrition is not only eating light vegetable dishes, but also the way in which we eat meals – careful and slow eating. Food should be chewed with calm and attention (15 to 20 times for each bite). We should focus only on the food and never watch TV or read the newspaper at the time. A short intention or prayer to thank for the meal is very important before eating.

Celebrate joy
A joyful person has unfathomable amounts of life force. We can see this wonderful energy in children who can enjoy life with all their bodies and souls. The joy of life, the joy of what happens in our lives, brings good mood, and thus more strength for further challenges and experiences.

Look into the heart
Empathy, or compassion, is a trait that helps to understand others. However, it is different from pity, which puts the other person below us. We are equal in feelings and emotions. Empathy is a beautiful feature of our heart and a bridge to build closeness with others.

Nurture gratitude

Gratitude is the expression of appreciation to God, the universe or fate for what is happening in your life. By cultivating it every day, you focus on seeing your own agency and the good that happens to you. By showing gratitude for what you receive from others, you deepen your relationship with them. You also give them a clear sign of what is important to you and that you see the good that they bring to you. Could there be a better incentive for further intimacy?

Create understanding

Understanding is knowledge that everything is exactly as it should be, which comes not from the mind, but from the heart. Understanding yourself gives you peace and vitality, understanding the people around you is an invaluable gift you can give them, understanding the world that surrounds you is a step to build joy and acceptance of your life.

<u>Exercise I:</u>
Write down the above litany and put it in a visible place, so that you can cultivate it in yourself everyday.

<u>Exercise II:</u>
Take a close look at what your life looks like as regards all the above points and figure out how to implement these principles.

<u>Example</u>
Being present in the moment – try setting a reminder in your phone at different times of the day saying: „Breathe. How do I feel?". Taking a few deep breaths will make you come back to being in the moment, and answering questions about feelings will show you what you need most at the moment.

Mindful eating – at the start of a particular meal try to focus on small bites and extend the time you spend on eating.

Workbook 4

Your Guide to Positive Life

12. THE NEED FOR LOVE AND THE LANGUAGE OF LOVE ACCORDING TO CHAPMAN

Gary Chapman, an American therapist and author of numerous books on relationships, shares his theory that strategies to meet the need for love can be divided into five groups, which he called the five languages of love. These are:

1. Words of appreciation and support
This is simply expressing love in words. It can be manifested by talking about what we like about the other person or why we enjoy being with them. It also includes verbal appreciation and celebration of their successes together.

2. Time spent together
The so-called „quality time" devoted to being with another person includes listening to what is important to them, sharing their passions or activities that make them happy (going to the cinema, going to the mountains, inviting them to a cafe).

3. Gifts
It is a pleasure to give presents to loved ones, but also to receive them. Remember that this is not about expensive material objects. The most important thing is the message the gift delivers: „I want to make you happy", „I know you and I know what is important to you".

4. Life enriching activities
These are various things, big and small, that can be done for another person, e.g. brewing tea and bringing it to bed, or doing some sort of chore for them.

5. Touch
This is physical tenderness, such as hugging, patting, holding hands, dancing, sexual activities. Why am I quoting Chapman's concepts here?

Recognizing which language of love we use and which our loved ones do is the basis for building relationships. Imagine that your basic language of love is touch. You expect it and you use it yourself, for example when you hug your friends in greeting.

However, your friends don't know they are important to you! Why? Their language of love is quality time spent together, so they arrange to go for a walk or to talk to you. However, you are not the person who initiates meetings. Do you see how much anxiety this can bring into your relationship? In this *Guide*, I want to show you how to find peace in your life!

If you know each other's languages of love, you will be able, for example, to write on your calendar a reminder to call and propose a meetup, and they will remember that when something good happens in your life, the biggest sign of love will be a hug, not saying „Congratulations".

How to find your love language?
Above all, I encourage you to read Chapman's books, but if you want to take a shortcut then you can find many websites where you can take a free test. Encourage those you really want to show your love to do so too.

Your Guide to Positive Life

13. YOUR INNER CRITIC

Your inner critic often causes shame and a sense of inadequacy. It can also cause self-doubt and undermine one's faith in their own abilities. It's a voice of anxiety in your heart. Do you know these thoughts? „I'm hopeless". „I can't do anything and I will certainly fail". „I'm fat and ugly".

The reason is the lack of unconditional love and acceptance from the people we love. If our loved ones show us love only when we meet their expectations, we learn that we can only achieve love by being perfect. They do not necessarily do it deliberately. However, it causes thoughts such as: „I have to meet the expectations of others to be loved", „I can't show that I make mistakes, because people will reject me."

This is one of the reasons for the lack of self-confidence, low self-esteem, constant shame of who you are. Diagnose all these problems in yourself, see in depth what they are and if you have the opportunity, speak honestly with those you love. Make sure that you show them unconditional love and tell them if you are afraid that you may lose their love because of „what ifs".

Exercise I:
Awareness is the first step to recognizing and releasing your inner critic. Identify the situation that may have caused an inner critic to surface.

Exercise II:
Replace overly critical thoughts with more specific statements. Change your pessimistic thoughts into a more rational and realistic ones.

Przykład
Replace „hopeless at cooking" with „I cooked a dinner that I didn't like on Wednesday, but today I made a delicious breakfast".
„I never get it right" - this thought often appears when we start doing something new and difficult. For example, if you are lear-

ning to dance and got your steps wrong for the third time, replace this thought with a statement of what actually took place, like „I got the steps wrong". When you do so, another thought will come: „what can I do to dance well?".

„Never" and „always" are two of the words blocking communication – including internal dialogue. They don't bring anything good, so throw them out of your dictionary.

Exercise III:
Every time a negative thought appears in your head, try to change it to a realistic description of the situation (example above), and if possible, look for positive statements.

Example
Going back to our example of erroneous dance steps. You can create some positive thoughts from a simple mistake that is typical for all beginners:

„I made a mistake, I remember that in the last class I also needed time to properly dance the new choreography. Now I dance it flawlessly, so I will definitely be able to do so with these steps".

„I still have so many things to learn, I can't wait to master this choreography".

Initially, this change of mindset may seem artificial and strange to you, but the more often you practice it, the more natural it will become for you to see the bright sides of your life. And from there, it's only one step to allow peace and joy into it!

Your Guide to Positive Life

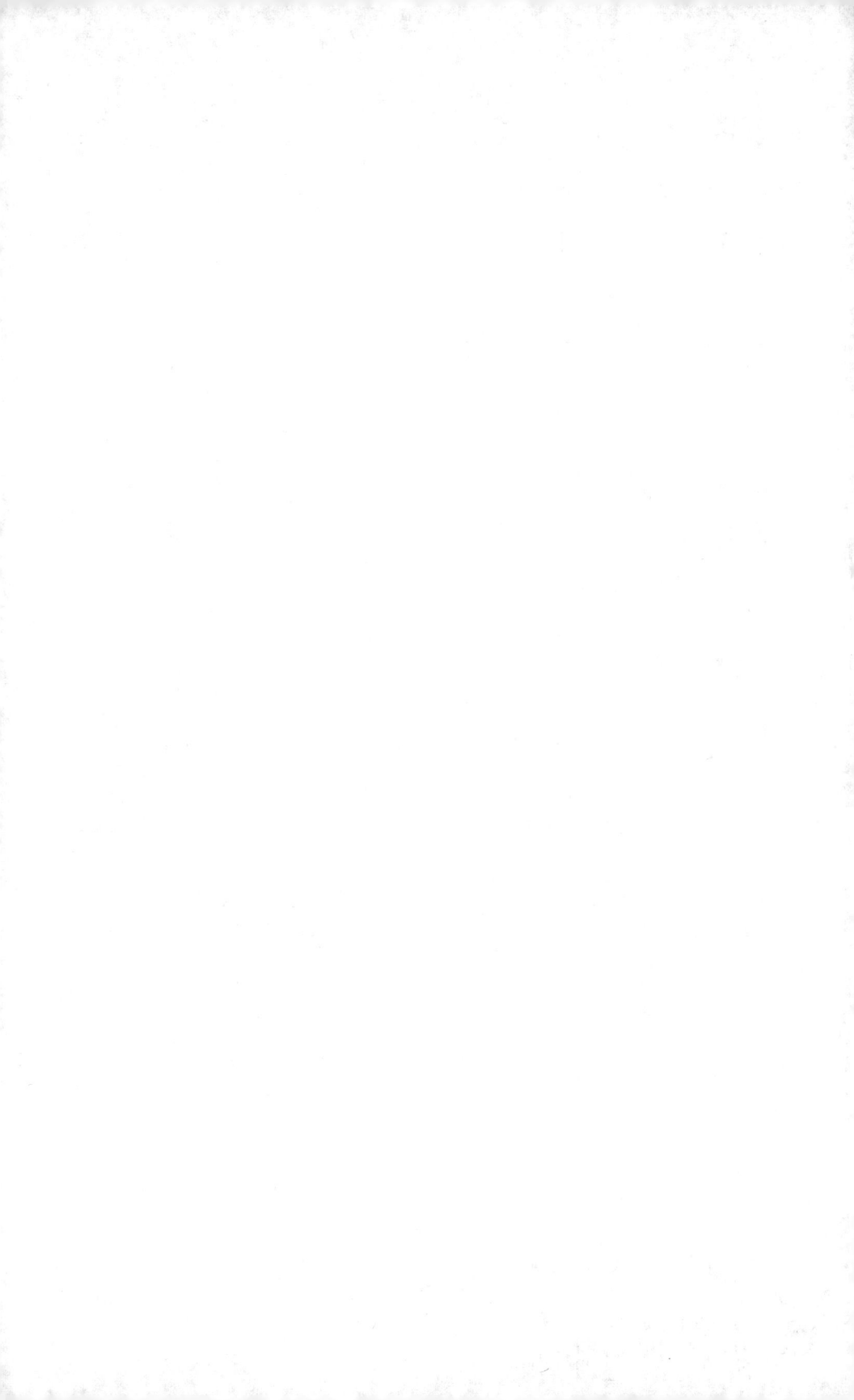

www.ingramcontent.com/pod-product-compliance
Lightning Source LLC
Chambersburg PA
CBHW051413290426
44108CB00015B/2266